797,885 Books

are available to read at

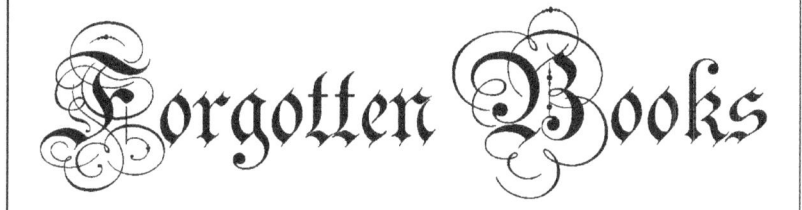

Forgotten Books

www.ForgottenBooks.com

Forgotten Books' App
Available for mobile, tablet & eReader

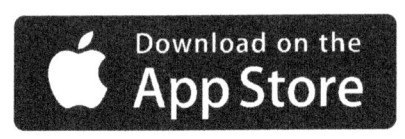

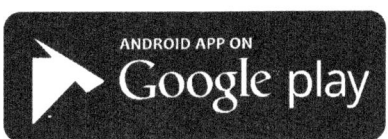

ISBN 978-1-332-24817-9
PIBN 10303977

This book is a reproduction of an important historical work. Forgotten Books uses state-of-the-art technology to digitally reconstruct the work, preserving the original format whilst repairing imperfections present in the aged copy. In rare cases, an imperfection in the original, such as a blemish or missing page, may be replicated in our edition. We do, however, repair the vast majority of imperfections successfully; any imperfections that remain are intentionally left to preserve the state of such historical works.

Forgotten Books is a registered trademark of FB &c Ltd.
Copyright © 2015 FB &c Ltd.
FB &c Ltd, Dalton House, 60 Windsor Avenue, London, SW19 2RR.
Company number 08720141. Registered in England and Wales.

For support please visit www.forgottenbooks.com

1 MONTH OF FREE READING

at
www.ForgottenBooks.com

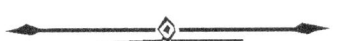

By purchasing this book you are eligible for one month membership to ForgottenBooks.com, giving you unlimited access to our entire collection of over 700,000 titles via our web site and mobile apps.

To claim your free month visit:
www.forgottenbooks.com/free303977

* Offer is valid for 45 days from date of purchase. Terms and conditions apply.

Similar Books Are Available from
www.forgottenbooks.com

Good Housekeeping
by Unknown Author

The Home Companion
A Guide and Counselor for the Household, by Unknown Author

Home Decoration
by Charles Franklin Warner

The Housekeeper's Handbook of Cleaning
by Sarah Josephine Macleod

Millionaire Households and Their Domestic Economy
With Hints Upon Fine Living, by Mary Elizabeth Carter

Successful Family Life on the Moderate Income
by Mary Hinman Abel

Convenient Houses, With Fifty Plans for the Housekeeper
by Louis H. Gibson

The Country Cottage
by George Llewellyn Morris

Furniture of the Olden Time
by Frances Clary Morse

A Syllabus of Household Management
by Mary Louise Furst

The Making of a Housewife
by Isabel Gordon Curtis

Household Engineering
Scientific Management in the Home, by Mrs. Christine Frederick

The Complete Housekeeper
by Emily Holt

Household Science
Or, Practical Lessons in Home Life, by Unknown Author

From Attic to Cellar
Or Housekeeping Made Easy, by Mrs. Elizabeth F. Holt

First Aid to the Young Housekeeper
by Christine Terhune Herrick

Housekeeping for Little Girls
by Olive Hyde Foster

Ethics of Household Economy
A Help to Inexperienced Wives and Discouraged Mothers, by E. McPherson-Parsons

Household Art
by Candace Wheeler

The Modern Household
by Marion Talbot

AN ACCOUNT

OF THE

Great Benefit of blowing Showers of FRESH AIR up thro' DISTILLING LIQUORS.

1. THE great Importance of having a sufficient Supply of fresh Water in Ships, has been the Occasion of many laudable Attempts to make Sea-water fresh and wholsome; but all the Attempts and Discoveries hitherto made, have laboured under this great and material Objection, *viz.* the great Quantity of Fuel that was necessary to distill, with a slow Progress, a small Quantity of Water, by any Methods of Distillation hi-

therto known. But I have lately happily, most unexpectedly, discovered an easy and effectual Method to distill great Quantities of Water with little Fuel; which I was led to by the following Incidents, *viz.* Mr. *Shipley*, Secretary of our Society, *for the Encouragement of Arts, Manufactures and Commerce*, brought me acquainted with Mr. *William Baily* of *Salisbury-Court*, the Author of many ingenious Contrivances; who shewed me, in a small Model of a Tin Vessel, a Method, by which he has happily increased the Force of the Engine to raise Water by Fire, *viz.* by lifting up some of the boiling Water, at every Stroke, by means of a conical Vessel, with small Holes in it, full of Tow; whereby the Quantity of the ascending Steam or Wreak was considerably increased. This led me to think, that a greater Quantity of Liquor might also by this Means be distilled; but on Trial I found the Increase to be only one twelfth Part, tho' considerable in the expanded Form of a Steam. Hence I was led to try what would be the Effect of causing an incessant Shower of Air to ascend thro' the

boiling

boiling Liquor in a Still; and this, to my Surprise, I found on Trial to be very considerable. There was another Circumstance also, which probably conduced to lead my Mind to this Thought, *viz.* About six Months before, Mr. *Littlewood*, a Shipwright at *Chatham*, came thence purposely to communicate to me an ingenious Contrivance of his, soon to sweeten stinking Water, by blowing a Shower of fresh Air thro' a Tin Pipe full of small Holes, layed at the Bottom of the Water. By this means, he told me, he had sweetened the stinking Bilge Water in the Well of some Ships; and also a But of stinking Water in an Hour, in the same manner as I blew Air up thro' Corn and Gunpowder, as mentioned in the Book on *Ventilators*.

2. The Method, which I used to blow Showers of Air up thro' the distilling Water, was by means of a flat round Tin Box, six Inches Diameter, and an Inch and half deep; which is placed at the Bottom of the Still, on four Knobs or Feet half Inch high, to make room for the Liquor to spread over the whole Bottom of the

Still, that the Heat of the Fire may come at it. In larger Stills this Box must be proportionably larger, and have higher Feet. And whereas the Mouth of the Still is too narrow, for the Tin Box to enter, which Box ought to be within two Inches as wide as the Bottom of the Still; therefore the Box may be divided into two Parts, with a Hinge at one Edge or Side, and a Clasp at the other, to fix it together, when in the Still. This Box must be of Copper for distilling Sea-wawater; mine was made of Tin for other Liquors also. The Air-pipe, which passes thro' the Head of the Still, will help to keep the Air-box from moving to and fro by the Motion of the Ship; or, if that should not be found sufficient, 3 or 4 small Struts may be fixed to the Sides of the Air-box. They must reach to the Sides of the Still. The Cover and Sides of the Air-box were punched full of very small Holes, one fourth Inch distant from each other, and about the twentieth part of an Inch in Diameter. On the Middle of the Cover or Lid of this Air-box, was fixed a Nosil more than half Inch wide, which

was

was fitted to receive, to put on, and take off the lower End of a Tin Pipe, which was twenty Inches long, and passed thro' a Hole in the Head of the Still: four Inches of the upper end of this Pipe were bent to a Crook, almost at a right Angle to the upright Stem, in order thereby to unite the Crook to the widened Nose of a Pair of Kitchen double Bellows, by means of a short Leathern Pipe of Calves-skin. See Fig. 1st. This Tin Air-box, and many more of them for other Persons, were made by Mr. *Tedway*, Tinman, over-against the *Meuse-Gate, Charing-Cross*.

3. THE double Bellows were bound fast to a Frame, at the upper Part of the Iron Nose, and at the lower Handle, in order the more commodiously to work them. And that the upper Half of the double Bellows may duly rise and fall, in order to cause a constant Stream of Air; (besides the usual contracting spiral Springs within side) several flat Weights of Lead must be layed on the upper Part of the Bellows, near the Handle, with a Hole in their Middle, to fix them on an upright Iron Pin fastened on the

Bel-

Bellows: That by this Means the Weights may the more commodiously be put on or taken off. For, according to the different Depths of the Liquor in the Still, so will the Force of the included Air, against the upper Board of the Bellows, be more or less. Thus, supposing the Depth of the Water in the Still to be twelve Inches; from the Surface of the depressed Water in the Air Box; then the Pressure of the included Air against the upper Part of the Bellows, will be equal to that of a Body of Water a Foot deep, and as broad as the inner Surface of that Board. It will, therefore, be requisite, to add or take off Weights, according to the different Depths of the Water in the Still, at different Periods of the same Distillation. The Bellows must be proportionable to the Size of the Still, but need not be very large. Wherever the Stills are fixed in Ships, the Air may be conveyed to them from the Bellows, either thro' a small leathern Pipe, distended with Spiral Coiles of Wyre, or thro' Bamboo Canes, or broad small wooden Pipes, like hollow fishing Rods.

4. When I first distilled in this ventilating Way, in order to estimate, what the Difference might be in the Quantity distilled, by that or the common Method, I tried both Ways, by receiving the distilled Liquor into a Quarter of a Pint Glass, estimating the Times, by a Pendulum beating Seconds. Where I found, to my Surprise, that sometimes three times more was distilled by Ventilation than by the usual Way: But finding Inequalities in the small Quantities thus distilled, in order the more fully and assuredly to ascertain the true Proportion there was in the two Methods of distilling, I put three Gallons of Water into the Still; and, when it boiled, put on the Still-head, and fixed its Nose to the Worm-tub Pipe; which Tub was full of cold Water. When it had distilled for an Hour, the Receiver was instantly taken away. And on measuring the distilled Water, found it to be two Quarts and 45 cubick Inches by a Glass divided into cubick Inches. And a Gallon containing 282 cubick or solid Inches, this Quantity of distilled Water, which

was

was 186 cubick Inches, is $\frac{1}{17}$th Part of a Gallon.

5. THEN, filling the Still as full of Water as before, and when it began to boil, fixing the Head to the Still and Worm-tub, which was full of cold Water; there was diſtilled in an Hour, with conſtantly blowing Showers of freſh Air up thro' the ſtilling Liquors, five Quarts, leſs by ſeven cubick Inches, which is 345.5ths cubick Inches; that is, little leſs than the double of the Quantity that is diſtilled in the uſual Way. In ſeveral other Diſtillations of a Quart at a Time, I found the Quantity diſtilled by Ventilation, to be more than the double of that in the uſual Way. So that the Quantity by Ventilation, may at a Medium be eſtimated the double of the uſual Diſtillation. It is the well known Property of moving Air, to carry along with it a conſiderable Quantity of adjoining Vapour, as alſo of falling Water to carry much Air down along with it.

6. IT is to be hoped therefore, that ſo conſiderable an Increaſe in the Quantity diſtilled,

diftilled, will be of great Benefit to Navigation, as it may be done in lefs Time and with lefs Fire.

7. In the Account of Mr. *Appleby*'s Procefs, for making Sea-water frefh, which is publifhed by Order of the Lords of the Admiralty in the Gazette of *Jan.* 22, 1754, it is faid that a Still which contains 20 Gallons of Water will diftill 60 Gallons in ten Hours with little more than one Bufhel of Coals; and therefore 120 Gallons in 20 Hours, with little more than two Bufhels of Coals. And by Ventilation 240 Gallons, or a Tun; and 24 Gallons may be diftilled in twenty Hours, making an Allowance for the times of heating thofe Stills full of cold Water; and a Still fomething larger and wider, will diftill a Tun in 24 Hours; which will more than fuffice for a fixty Gun Ship with 400 Men, whofe Provifion of Water for four Months is about 110 Tuns. And larger Ships may either have proportionably larger Stills, or elfe two of them. As for Merchant-Ships with few Men, a fmall Still will be fufficient.

8. The

8. The second sized Stills contain 10 Gallons, and will produce 60 Gallons in 20 Hours, with half the above-mentioned Fuel; and by Ventilation 120 Gallons.

9. The least Stills contain five Gallons, and will produce 32 Gallons in 20 Hours; and by Ventilation 64 Gallons in 20 Hours.

10. I have seen some of these Stills at Messrs. *Steel* and *Stephens*, over-against *Mercers-Chapel*, in *Cheapside*, which have been made for this Purpose. There are Holes in the Feet of the Iron Frame or Stove to skrew them down to the Deck. They were fixed at the Fore-castle before the Mast in King *Charles* the Second's time, when they thought they had discovered the Way to distill Sea-water, free from the noxious Spirit of Salt, and from the nauseous bittern Taste. Or, if it be thought proper, one Part of the Ship's Boiler may be made use of, by adapting a Still-head to it.

11. Now

FRESH WATER *at* SEA. 13

11. Now suppofing a Still to contain 25 Gallons, and that four Parts in five of it, *viz.* 20 Gallons are diftilled off: then, in order to diftill *a Tun,* or 210 *Gallons,* the Still muft be emptied, cleanfed and refilled eleven times; and if the whole be done in 24 Hours, full 16 of thofe Hours will be taken up in diftilling at the rate of a Gallon in about four Minutes and half; and the remaining eight Hours of the 24, being divided into 11 equal Parts, they will be each near 44 Minutes to empty and cleanfe the Still, to refill it, and give the Sea-water a proper boiling diftilling Heat: whether this can be done in fo fhort a Time, muft be known by Experience, and ought therefore firft to be tried at Land.

12. Doctor *Butler,* in his lately publifhed Method of *procuring Frefh Water at Sea,* propofes the pouring in more Seawater into the Still, thro' a Funnel fixed in a fmall Hole in the Head or Upper-part of the Still, when more than half the former Water is diftilled off; by which means the Water in the Still will foon acquire a diftilling

ling Heat; and this to be repeated several times; but then it will be requisite to add each time more Chalk, in such Proportion as shall be found requisite. It will be well to try this Method in hopes thereby to increase the Quantity of Water that is distilled. The Hole in the Head, or Upper-part of the Still, is to be stopped with a small Plate of Copper, so fixed as to turn to and fro over the Hole.

13. DOCTOR *Butler* used capital Soap Lees, in the Proportion of a Wine Quart to 15 Gallons of Sea-water, which sufficed for four or five times repeated Pourings in of more Sea-water into the Still. But as I have found that a small Quantity of Chalk has the same good Effect, and is cheaper, and more easily to be had, it is therefore preferable to Soap Lees.

14. WHEN there is a Fire in the Cook-room, the Sea-water might be ready heated to put into the Still, without any additional Expence of Fuel, in the following Manner, which I shall here describe; tho' I think it probable that it will not be put

in practice; yet, as farther Improvements may possibly hereafter be made in it, and as it may be of use in some Cases, at Land at least, I shall here give an Account of it, *viz.*

15. About the Year 1718, Mr. *Schmetou*, a *German* Gentleman, got a Patent here for heating great Quantities of Water, with little Expence of Fuel, which he then shewed me. Having fixed a spiral Iron Worm-pipe, in such a Brick Stove or Chimney as Women heat their Irons in, thereby causing the Water to run from a Vessel, thro' the Worm-pipe, several Feet Length round, in the Fire. About 30 Years after I acquainted Mr. *Cramond* of *Twickenham* with this, as hoping it might be of Benefit in distilling Sea-water. Upon which he procured such a spiral Iron Worm-pipe, which was about twenty Feet long, and six-tenths Inch Diameter; the Diameter of the spiral Coile was about fourteen Inches.

16. This I fixed in a Brick Stove in my Garden, with its upper End fixed to a

Vessel, which contained 45 Gallons of Water. I found the Event of this first Trial to be as follows, *viz*. When the Water run full Bore, at the rate of a Gallon in 17 Seconds, the Heat of the Water was found, by a mercurial Thermometer held in the Stream, at the lower End of the Pipe, to be 80 Degrees above the freezing Point, 180 Degrees being the Heat of boiling Water. When by means of a Turn-cock, a Gallon of Water was two Minutes in running, then the Heat was 140. At which Rate the 45 Gallons would be an Hour and half in running thro' the Iron-pipe; at which Rate 25 Gallons will run thro' in 50 Minutes, with so considerable a Degree of Heat; and if it was an Hour running, the Heat would approach still nearer to a boiling Heat, when first put into the Still, which would forward the Distillation if wanted.

17. I PUMPED the heated Water up again into the upper Vessel; and thus continued to circulate the heating Water, till its Heat was 160 Degrees in the upper Vessel, *viz*. within 20 Degrees, or one-ninth

ninth of boiling, the Heat requiſite for plentiful Diſtillation. I was in hopes that if the Water in the upper Veſſel could have been brought to a due Degree of Heat, and a Still-head were fixed on it, with its cooling Worm-tub, then Water might have been diſtilled in Ships, by having the Iron Worm-pipe fixed in the Chimney of the Cook-room: But I found, that when the Heat of the Water in the upper Veſſel was 160 Degrees, *viz.* within one-ninth of boiling; then in running through the Iron Worm-pipe again, it was ſo over-heated, as to expand in the Pipe, into an exploſive Vapour, which hindered the running of the Water. However I thought it not improper to give an Account of this Attempt, notwithſtanding it failed. Not knowing whether this Method of heating Water, may not in ſome Caſes, at Land at leaſt, be of uſe, thereby to ſave, in ſome degree, both Fuel and Time: Perhaps an Iron Worm-pipe of a larger Bore might do better.

18. THE Waſte of Fuel will be leſs in proportion to the Quantity diſtilled in
large,

large, than in small Stills; and the wider the Still-head is, so much the more Liquor will be distilled, and more with a Worm-tub than without it. The Worm-tub may be so covered, as to prevent the flowing over of the Water by the Motion of the Ship.

19. It is of great Importance to take care to keep all Parts of the Still clean, that there may be no Rust or Verdigrease in the Copper, which will occasion Vomiting.

20. If it be necessary, the better to close the Joining of the Still-head, it may be done with a Lute or Paste made of a Mixture of powdered Chalk and Meal, wetted with Salt-water.

21. Now that several effectual Means are discovered, to make distilled Sea-water wholsome, and also to distill it in much greater Quantity in the same Still, in the same Time, and with nearly the same Quantity of Fuel; it is reasonable to believe, that it will be of great Benefit to Navi-

Navigation, not only in saving much stowage room, for other important Purposes; but also in procuring fresh sweet wholsome Water, instead of stinking putrid Water, hitherto used; which must needs have a Tendency to promote that putrid Distemper, the Scurvy. And if withal due Care be taken, to exchange for fresh Air the putrid close confined Air of Ships, which has occasioned the Death of Millions of Mankind; then Navigation will become remarkably more healthy, and, with little more Danger to Health and Life, than at Land, except from Storms.

22. Now supposing, that in a sixty Gun Ship, the 110 Tuns of Water, for four Months use, were distilled at the Expence of three Bushels of Coals to a Tun, this would consume nine Chaldrons of Coals: And as a Chaldron of Coals weighs about a Tun and half; hence it appears that Coals will distill about eight times their Quantity of Water. And the 110 Tuns of Water weighing (at the Rate of 2240 Pounds to the Tun) 138 Tuns; and the nine Chaldrons of Coals weighing thirteen Tuns and half,

half, that is 94 Tuns and half less than the 110 Tuns of Store-water; and allowing twenty-four Tuns and half for the Still, Water-casks, and Coals, there will be 70 Tuns Weight of Stowage saved thereby for *other Uses*. Or if some Tuns of Storewater are carried by way of Precaution, which it will be advisable to do, especially at first, till they can be assured, by repeated Experience, what Quantity can be depended upon by Distillation; even then about half the Tunnage will be saved, which will be a very material Advantage.

23. Tho' when the distilling Liquor runs from the Bottom of the Worm-pipe, thro' a long Pipe fixed to it, the Waste by the ventilating rushing Air, is not great when the Water in the Worm-tub is not hot; yet the following Precaution, if needful, may be used, in distilling by Ventilation, *viz.* to fix at the lower End of the Worm-pipe, by means of a wooden Fawcet, a small Cask for a Receiver; the Fawcet to enter the upper side of the Head of the Cask, and in order to give a free Passage for the great Quantity of ventilating

ing Air to pass off, and withal at the same time to prevent the escaping of much moist Vapour with it, it will be proper to fix at the Bung-hole a long upright Pipe of Wood, or of any Metal. I used a Gun-barrel four Feet and a half long; through which some small Degree of moist Vapour escaped; as appeared by the Dampness of a Piece of Paper, fixed at a little Distance above the Mouth of the Gun-barrel. This Vapour became visible, and much increased, when the Water in the Worm-tub was very hot; at which Time, less is distilled into the Cask-receiver; then also there is more Danger of the Spirit of Salt arising. And it was observable, that the Water in the Worm-pipe Vessel heated much sooner by Ventilation, than in the common Way of distilling. For which Reason that Water ought to be changed so much the oftener, which can easily be done at Sea. The Cocks also at the Side of the Worm-tub ought to be large, in order to let the hot Water off the faster.

24. But tho' the Water in the Worm-tub was sooner heated by Ventilation, be-

cause a double Quantity of hot Steam passed thro' it, more than passed thro' it in equal Times in the common Way of distilling; yet in the usual Way of Distillation the Liquor in the Still is hotter, with equal Fire, as is evident by its aptness to boil over thro' the Worm-pipe; whereas in the ventilating Way it did not boil over, notwithstanding a very hot Fire was purposely made for a Trial. The continual Streams of ascending fresh Air, not only in some Degree abating the Heat of the Water; but also incessantly carrying off the more rarefied Particles of the Water, which, when expanded into a repelling State, do thereby cause the overflowing Ebullition of the Water. On which Account it is probable, that less Spirit of Salt is formed and raised by Ventilation than without it As also on account of the fresh Air ascending, not from the Bottom of the Still, where is the greatest Plenty of Salt, especially towards the latter End of each Distillation; but about three Inches from the Bottom, *viz.* principally from the many Holes at the Surface of the Air-box.

25. A<small>ND</small>

25. And whereas the Quantity raised from the Still, and distilled into the Cask-receiver, cannot be seen; the proper Quantity to be distilled in each Distillation, may with great Accuracy be known, by having a well closed Pewter Bottle of the Size of about half a Pint, with a Brass Wyre as big as a Goose Quill fixed to it, the Wyre to pass thro' the Receiver-cask, near the Bung-hole, which the floating Pewter Bottle will raise up, till the Marks on the Wyre appear just above the Cask. I made use of a Glass Viol for this Purpose. This Wyre will rise and fall freely, notwithstanding the Motion of the Ship, if it passes not only thro' the Wood of the Cask, but also thro' a metaline Pipe two or three Inches long, fixed in that Hole. And it will be known by the simmering or boiling Noise of the Water in the Still, whether it is hot enough to distill; for the running of the Water into the Receiver-cask cannot be seen

26. As it might be suspected, that more Spirit of Salt would be raised, and distilled

over in the ventilating Way, than without it; having procured 18 Gallons of Sea-water by the *Margate* Hoy, which was taken up at some Distance from the Shore, I put three Gallons of this Sea-water, as soon as I had received it, into the Still; and when it began to distill, Air was blown up thro' it. For some Time, as is usual, in the Distillation of Sea-water; no Spirit of Salt arose; but after distilling some Time longer, there were very weak whitish Clouds, with Drops of Solution of Silver in Aqua-fortis, as in the common Way of distilling. Hence we see, that Ventilation does not increase the Quantity of Salt, but rather probably somewhat decreases it, for the Reasons above given, N° 24.

27. I DISTILLED three Gallons of Sea-water, which had stunk and became sweet again; when about ten Quarts of it had been distilled off, then there began to be very weak whitish Clouds with Solution of Silver, but none with Solution of Mercury; which shows the Water to be hitherto good, agreeably to what I formerly had found to be the good Effect of distilling

Sea-water, which had putrified, and become sweet again; of which I published an Account in the Year 1739. But when I continued the Distillation on, a quarter of an Hour longer, *viz.* till there was but a Pint of Water remaining in the Still, and the Salts were incrusted on its Sides, up near three Inches from the Bottom, and lay in Heaps at the Bottom of the Still, then the distilled Liquor had whitish Clouds in it, with the Solution of Mercury in Aqua-fortis. From this Distillation we see, that Putrefaction, by dissolving the bittern Salt and Bitumen, into very minute Parts, qualified them to combine with the more fixed common Salt, so as to detain them from rising in Distillation.

28. I DISTILLED three Gallons of Sea-water, with the Proportion of six Ounces of Mr. *Appleby*'s Lapis Infernalis, and six Ounces of calcined Bones to 20 Gallons of Sea-water, as he directs. This Water lathered well with Soap, and boiled Peas well.

29. I DISTILLED also some Sea-water with half an Ounce of Stone Lime to a Gallon,

Gallon, from the *Clee* Hills in *Herefordshire*, which having been preserved ten Months in a Firkin, had slacked to dry Powder. This distilled Water did also lather well with Soap, and boiled Peas well; which proves that the Lime, which is a fixed Body, does not distill over with the Water. Since I made this Distillation, General *Oglethorpe* informed me, that his Father, Sir *Theophilus*, told him, that Lime was one of the Ingredients, of what he and the rest of the Patentees, in *Charles* the Second's time, called the Cement, with which they made distilled Sea-water wholsome.

30. I DISTILLED also some Sea-water with the like Proportion of powdered Chalk, which boiled Peas well, and was better tasted than the Waters distilled with Lapis Infernalis or Lime. I distilled also some Sea-water with an Ounce of Chalk to a Gallon, but found no Difference in the Taste of this, and that which had but half an Ounce of Chalk to a Gallon: So that half an Ounce of Chalk to a Gallon of Water will be sufficient; but where the

the Sea-water is falter, or more bituminous, more Chalk may be added if needful

31. Dr. *Alston* of *Edinburgh*, in the Preface to the Second Edition of his Dissertation on Quick-lime and Lime-water, says, that " the like Effect was found in " distilling Sea-water with Lime, that it " neither precipitated a Solution of Silver " in Aqua-fortis, nor a Solution of cor" rosive Sublimate in Water, nor did it " form a Pellicle of various Colours on " its Surface, as did the Water distilled " by Mr. *Appleby*'s Process." And I find, Page 35 of my Book on this Subject, that Lime of Oyster-shells had the same good Effect, but required two Distillations; I might then use too small a Quantity of that Lime. Hence it is probable, that the Chalk, the Lime, the Lime in the Lapis Infernalis, and the Lime in Dr. *Butler*'s Soap-lees, seize on and fix not only the bittern Salt, but also the Bitumen of the Sea-water, as we learn from the like Effect in the Purification of the Salt of Hartshorn. That the saline Spirit arises chiefly

from

from the bittern Salt, and not from the more perfect Sea-salt, is probable from hence, *viz.* when I distilled three Gallons of common Water, made as salt as Sea-water with common Salt; no Spirit of Salt arose, even tho' the Distillation was carried so far as to leave the Salt, tho' very damp, to lie in Heaps, and it was incrusted on the Sides of the Still, for about three Inches from the Bottom.

32. It is a considerable further Advantage, that Water thus distilled by Ventilation, being thereby repleat and freshened with Air, has for present Use a more agreeable Taste, than Water distilled without Ventilation, which requires the standing a longer Time to have its more disagreeable adust Taste go off. And as the volatile Oil of Pepper-mint does rise on the Wings of the ventilating Air during the Distillation; so also may that Part of the Bitumen, which is volatilized by Heat; as also the volatile urinous Salts of the Sea water, which arises from animal Substances, be sublimed in the same Manner.

33. It

Fresh Water at SEA. 29

33. It was observable, that the Water distilled fast, even tho' the Water in the Still was below the Surface of the Tin Air-box, thro' which the greatest Part of the ascending Shower of Air rushed. Hence the ventilating Air, in ascending among the Vapours, carries them off fast. Hence it is to be suspected, that this Method of Ventilation will not do well for simple Waters, or fermented vinous Spirits; because they being very volatile, much of them may be carried off in Waste.

34. It was observable, that in these Distillations of Sea-water, no whitish Clouds appeared on dropping in Solution of corrosive Mercury, not even when considerably more than four Parts in five of the Water had been distilled over. And it was the same with the Mixture of Lapis Infernalis, Lime, and Chalk; whence it is probable, that the Lime and Chalk seize on and fix the more volatile bittern Salt, as does also the Lime in the Lapis Infernalis. And it is well known, that Sugar, that sweet Salt, cannot be made without Lime, on which, as its Centre of Union, it fixes and granulates.   35. And

35. AND whereas with a Solution of Silver in Aquafortis, which was much weakened and diluted with Water, there appeared a faint Degree of whitish Cloud, in all the above-mentioned Distillations, tho' not with the stronger Solution of Mercury till the Distillation was carried on, much beyond four Parts in five of the Water in the Still; when both Solutions caused remarkably white Clouds, especially the Solution of Mercury; which indicates the Quantity of the Spirit of Salt which was raised during the former part of the Distillation to be exceeding small, since it could not seize on, nor disengage the Aqua-fortis from the stronger Solution of Mercury, tho' it did in a very small Degree in the weak Solution of Silver, so as to let loose a very little of the Silver, which thereby caused the faint Clouds. When a Drop of the Solution of Mercury was dropped into the distilled Water, after a Drop of the Solution of Silver, it resorbed the Silver Cloud, and made the Water clear, by means of the great Proportion of acid Aqua-fortis that was in it.

36. Now

Fresh Water at Sea. 31.

36. Now in order to make some Estimate of the very small Quantity of Spirit of Salt in these several distilled Waters, I dropped a Drop of the Solution of Silver into an Ounce, or 480 Grains of pure Rain Water, which gave no Clouds; but on dropping in a Drop of Sea-water, which weighed a Grain, the white Clouds were strong. And since Sea-water can dissolve nine times more Salt than it has in it; therefore, supposing the Drop to be so fully impregnated with Salt, then the Salt would be the 480th Part of the Ounce of Water. But as there is nine times less Salt, therefore the Proportion of the Quantity of Spirit of Salt will be but the 4320th Part. And how much less must be the Proportion of Salt in these distilled Waters, which is not sufficient to make a sensible Impression on Solution of Mercury, and but a faint one on much diluted Solution of Silver. Such distilled Sea-water will not therefore, probably be unwholsome; almost all Spring-waters have some Degree of Salt in them: But if there were more of the Spirit of Salt, a

very

very small Quantity of Pot-ash, or Pearl-ashes, or Salt of Tartar, combined with it, will turn it into common Salt, the Quantity of which would be extremly little

37. It may be well to be provided in Ships with some Silver dissolved in Aquafortis, mixed with pure Rain-water, or distilled fresh Water, in the Proportion of sixty Drops to an Ounce of the Water; tho' it is probable, it may seldom be wanted, unless in some doubtful Cases, when the Taste may not be accurate enough to perceive, whether there be any Spirit of Salt in the distilled Water.

38. Since double the usual Quantity of Vapour may by Way of Ventilation be carried off, common Salt may thus be made much sooner, cheaper, and better; because as there is much less Fire used; so proportionably, less of the fine acid Spirit of the Salt, in which its Virtue consists, will be evaporated away: For it is well known, that the Salt is best which has undergone the least Action of Fire in making.

39. This

39. This more speedy Method of evaporating will also be useful, in making many other Evaporations; as in making Pot-ash, &c.

40. But some are apprehensive, that this great Improvement in Distilling, may be of ill Consequence in making those destructive Spirits cheaper, which are already but too cheap. Had not the Improvement been of great Benefit to Mankind in many other Respects, I should have been far, very far, from endeavouring after it, or discovering it. But should the Event be to make those Spirits cheaper, and consequently, by spreading farther, more destructive, the consequence of that will be, that the increased raging Devastation will the sooner necessarily rouse the Nations to put a Stop to what must be done hereafter; for if the Ravages continue increasing, as they have done for sixty Years past, the human Species must needs not only be greatly debased, but even in great measure diminished and destroyed. And yet none of the Nations, whose very Vi-

tals are thereby confuming and deftroying, endeavour to put any Stop to it, except the Heads of the native Indians in *North-America*, who have long repeatedly intreated the *English* to fell them no Rum; which is as effectually extirpating of them, as the Hornet did the unfubdued remainder of the *Canaanites*.

41. IF Mankind, inftead of receiving and entertaining this Peft with almoft univerfal Applaufe and Approbation, could prevail with themfelves to be in earneft to ufe Means to deliver themfelves from it; then much might be done towards it, by lowering and weakening all kind of fermented diftilled Spirits with Water, to a falutary Degree, as is now practifed in our Plantations in *America*, in making Punch fo weak, as not to be hurtful; which, when it was much ftronger, was well known to deftroy Multitudes. And where the like humane, wife, and laudable Practice has been ufed in Ships, it has had the fame happy falutary Effect.

42. WHAT

42. What Necessity or even Temptation can there be to be averse to the making them wholsome, instead of being venomous and destructive? and that not only of the Lives, but even of the Morals of Mankind. How much therefore does it behove all, who have any Concern for the Honour and Dignity of their own kindred Species, any Indignation at its being thus debased and disgraced, any Bowels of Pity for the vast Multitudes, not less than a Million, that are yearly destroyed all over the World, by this moral as well as natural, and therefore worst of all Evils that ever befel unhappy Man; to use their utmost Endeavours to deliver Mankind from this Pest? But notwithstanding this astonishing Ravage and Destruction of the human Species, yet the unhappy unrelenting Nations of the World, seem as unconcerned about it, as if only so many Thousands, nay, Millions of Caterpillers or Locusts were destroyed thereby. Was there ever a more important Occasion to rouse the Indignation of Mankind? Can we be calm and undisturbed, when this mighty

Deſtroyer rears up its invenomed Head every where? The moſt zealous Advocates for Drams, even the unhappy beſotted Dramiſts themſelves, the prolonging of whoſe Lives, and whoſe real Welfare both here and hereafter, is hereby ſincerely intended, cannot find fault with this wellmeant Remonſtrance, in Defence of them, and of all Mankind, againſt this mighty Deſtroyer, from one who has long been labouring, and that not without Succeſs, in finding Means to preſerve Multitudes of Lives, by various Ways.

An Account of the great Benefit of VENTILATORS *in many Instances, in preserving the* HEALTH *and* LIVES *of People, in Slave and other Transport Ships.*

43. IT is to be hoped that the several Means here proposed for having fresh and sweet Water at Sea, will be of great Benefit in preserving the Health and Lives of Multitudes of that valuable and useful Part of Mankind, those who occupy their Business in great Waters; whose Welfare I have long had at heart, and endeavoured to promote by various Ways; especially by finding Means to procure them fresh salutary Air, instead of the noxious, putrid, close confined pestilential Air, which has destroyed Millions of Mankind in Ships. And it is to be hoped that by diligent Researches, farther and farther useful Discoveries will hereafter be made for the Benefit of Navigation.

44. THE following, as they are strong Proofs of the great Benefit and Usefulness

of Ventilators in Ships, so they also fully prove that they can most commodiously be fixed and worked in them, in contradiction to the vulgar, false, and groundless Notion, that they take up too much room, and are incommodious, and in a manner impracticable to be worked, whereas the Men are eager to work them; and many more Persons can be with Safety to their Health and Lives in a ventilated, than in an unventilated Ship; which fully obviates the Objection as to the Room they take up. In new and important Researches, the likeliest Way to succeed, is to pursue a Thought not only by imperfect and fallacious Reasonings, but when the Nature of the Thing requires it, with a proper Series of Trials and Experiments. Thus in the present Case, the principal Cause of the Sickness in Ships, is the noxious putrid Air; the obvious Remedy is the exchanging that foul Air for fresh, by effectual Means, which are seldom discovered by dwelling only on Objections, but are usually the Reward of repeated diligent, experimental Researches. Neither are we to be discouraged in these our Purſuits by ſome Diſappointments, for I have frequently found that they lead to the Thing ſought for: And by the like Clue of Reaſoning and Experimenting, there is the greateſt Probability that we ſhall ſucceed in another very important Reſearch, *viz.* the preſerving much longer from Decay the Timbers of Ships laid up in ordinary in Harbour: For as we are aſſured by daily Experience, that the Decay is wholly owing to damp, cloſe confined putrid corroding Air; ſo the only Remedy for this Evil, is the frequently changing the Air among the Timbers, by plentiful Ventilations; which we find by happy Experience, can be effected to ſuch a Degree, as give reaſonable Hopes, enough to encourage our farther Trials and Reſearches.

45. CAPTAIN *Thomſon* of the *Succeſs Frigate*, in his Letter to me dated *London*, Sept. 25, 1749, ſays, " That during
" the Ventilation, the Lower-deck Hatches
" were commonly kept cloſe ſhut; by
" which means the Air was drawn down
" into the Hold, from between Decks,
" thro' the Seams of the Ceiling, along the
" Timbers

"Timbers of the Ship; by which means we found the foul Air soon drawn off from between Decks. Our Rule for ventilating was for half an Hour every four Hours; but when the Ventilating was sometimes neglected for eight Hours together, then we could perceive, especially in hot Weather, a very sensible Difference by that short Neglect of it; for it would then take a longer Time to draw off the foul Air. Our general Rule was, to work the Ventilators till we found the Air from them sweet. We all agreed that they were of great Service; the Men being so sensible of the Benefit of them, that they required *no driving* to work that which they received so much Benefit by. We found this good Effect from Ventilation, that tho' there were near 200 Men on board, for almost a Year, yet I landed them all well in *Georgia*, notwithstanding they were pressed Men, and delivered me out of Goals, with Distempers upon them. This is what I believe but few Transports, or any other Ships, can brag of; nor did I ever meet the like Good-luck before;

"which

" which, next to Providence, I impute to
" the Benefit received by the Ventilators.
" It is to be remarked, that we who lay
" wind-bound, for four Months, with
" our Expedition Fleet, which foon after
" invaded *France*, were very healthy all
" the time, when they were very fickly in
" all the Ships of that Expedition.

46. " THIS certainly occafioned all kind
" of Grain Provifions to keep better and
" longer from Weevels, than otherwife
" they would have done; and other Kinds
" of Provifions received Benefit from the
" Coolnefs and Frefhnefs in the Air of
" the Ship, which was caufed by Ventila-
" tion."

47. MR. *Cramond* alfo informs me, that he found the good Effect of Ventilators on board a Slave-Ship of his with 392 Slaves, twelve of which were taken on board, juft before they failed from *Guinea*, ill of a Flux, which twelve all died; but the reft, with all the *Europeans* in the Ship, arrived well at *Buenos Ayres*.

The

The following is a Letter to me from Captain ELLIS, *viz.*

"SIR,

48. "COULD any thing increase the Pleasure I have in a literary Intercourse with you, it would be to find that it answered your End in promoting the public Good. The *Vis-inertiæ* of Mankind is not the only Difficulty you have had to encounter, but their Ignorance and Prejudices, which are almost insuperable. It is to your Perseverance and Resolution, that the little Progress you have made is due: Indeed I ought not to say little; for it is a great Step to have found the few that have Hearts good enough to relish your Plan, and Heads sufficiently clear to discern the most effectual Method of advancing it. It does Honour to those noble and other worthy Personages that join you in Acts of such extensive Humanity, as the Introduction of Ventilators to Hospitals, Prisons, Ships of War and Transport, &c. as they must necessarily render the Miseries of the first more supportable,

"and

" and the close and constant Confinement
" of the others less prejudicial and fatal to
" their Health and Life. It is to be la-
" mented that they are not more generally
" made use of; for, notwithstanding their
" Advantage is apparent and incontestable,
" it is scarce credible how few are to be
" found among the vast Number of Ships
" daily employed in carrying Passengers,
" Slaves, Cattle, and other perishable Com-
" modities. Those of your Invention,
" which I had, were of singular Service to
" us; they kept the Inside of the Ship cool,
" sweet, dry, and healthy: The Number
" of Slaves I buried was only six, and not
" one white Man of our Crew, (which
" was thirty-four) during a Voyage of 15
" Months; an Instance very uncommon.
" The 340 Negroes were very sensible of
" the Benefits of a constant Ventilation,
" and were always displeased when it was
" omitted: Even the Exercise had Advan-
" tages not to be despised among People
" so much confined. I must not, however,
" forget that Ventilation alone is insuffi-
" cient to keep Disorders out of Ships;
" for often Infections are brought aboard
" by

"by the Slaves, or others; and frequently
"Diseases are produced by feeding on bad
"or decayed Food, but oftener still by
"Insobriety; for I have ever remarked,
"that the immoderate Use of spirituous
"Liquors in warm Climates, is more per-
"nicious and fatal even than the Malig-
"nancy of the Air itself. In cold Coun-
"tries too, where I have had Experience,
"those Sailors, or others, who accustom-
"ed themselves to hard drinking, especi-
"ally of Drams, had the Scurvy in a ter
"rible Degree; whereas those who were
"temperate or sober, either escaped it en-
"tirely, or had it but moderately. The
"Effects of Drunkenness was still more
"discernable among the Indians adjoining
"our Settlements in *Hudson's-Bay*, who
"are a feeble, diminutive, chilly, indo-
"lent Set of People. On the contrary,
"those who come from the inland Parts
"(who are unused to drink Brandy) are
"brave, active, robust, and industrious.
"The same Difference is observable in the
"*Africans*, and perhaps among the Inha-
"bitants of most other Nations, did we at-
"tend to it. It was to the unusual Sobri-
"ety

" ety of my Crew, that I afcribed, in fome
" meafure, their uncommon Healthinefs;
" for Sailors breathe a purer Air, and en-
" joy more Exercife and Liberty, than
" Paffengers or Slaves; wherefore their
" Ailments are owing to bad or diforder-
" ly Living, as well as to unwholfome
" Air.

" Could I but fee the immoderate Ufe
" of fpirituous Liquors lefs general, and
" the Benefits of Ventilators more known
" and experienced, I might then hope to
" fee Mankind better and happier. I am,

" S I R,

" *Your moft obediens Servant*,

Briftol, Dec.
26, 1753.

HENRY ELLIS."

49. And, by the like good Conduct, in his next Voyage in the Year 1755, not one of 312 Slaves died; and all his 36 Sailors arrived alive and well at *Briftol*.

50. And the Earl of *Halifax* has often informed me of the great Benefit they found by the Ufe of Ventilators, in feve-
ral

ral *Nova Scotia* Transport-Ships, twelve to one more have been found to die in unventilated than in ventilated Ships. It is indeed a self-evident Thing, that the changing the foul Air frequently in Ships, in which there are many Persons, will be a means of keeping them in better Health than not doing it; which makes it the more astonishing that effectual Proposals to remedy so great an Evil, should be received with so much Coldness and Indifference by Mankind. They little consider that it is the high Degree of Putrefaction (that most subtile Dissolvent in Nature) which a foul Air acquires in long stagnating, which gives it that pestilential Quality, which causes what is called the Goal-Distemper. And a very small Quantity, or even Vapour of this highly attenuated Venom, like the Infection or Inoculation for the Small-pox, soon spreads its deadly Infection. Ought not Men therefore, from the common natural Principle of Self-Preservation, to use their utmost Endeavours to shun this pestilent Destroyer, by which Millions of Mankind have perished in Ships?

An Account of some Tryals to cure the ill Taste of MILK, *which is occasioned by the Food of* COWS, *either from Turnips, Cabbages, or autumnal Leaves,* &c. *Also to sweeten* STINKING-WATER, &c.

51. THIS Method of blowing Showers of Air up thro' Liquors, will be of considerable Use in several other Respects, as well as in Distillation, as appears by the following Trials, *viz.*

52. I HAVE been informed that it is a common Practice, to cure the ill Taste of Cream from the Food of Cows, by setting it in broad Pans over hot Embers or Charcoal, and continually stirring it, till scalding hot, and till cool again: But when I attempted to do this much sooner, and more effectually, by blowing Showers of Air up thro' it; I soon found it to be impracticable, by reason of its very great Degree of frothing up. The ill Taste must therefore be got out of the Milk, before it
is

is set for Cream; which I have been told, has been practised, and that with some benefit, by giving the Milk a scalding Heat, without stirring it.

53. *May* 22. I ventilated some ill tasted, new unheated Milk of a Cow which was purposely fed with Crow Garlick mixed with cut Grass. After 15 Minutes Ventilation the Taste was a little mended; in half an Hour's blowing it was something better. At the Hour's end it had the same Taste, but was sensibly better than the unventilated Milk. I was disappointed of an Opportunity to repeat the Experiment with Crow Garlick Milk, with a scalding Heat; it would then probably have been soon perfectly cured; as it is reasonable to believe from the Event of the following Experiments, *viz.*

54. *August* 23, four Quarts of ill tasted new Milk, from a Cow which had fed eighty-four Hours on Cabbage Leaves only, and drank during that Time very little Water; were put into a leaden Vessel, eight Inches in Diameter, and thirty Inches deep.

ches deep. The leaden Veſſel was heated in a large Boiler, and ſet into a Veſſel of hot Water; thereby to give the Milk a ſcalding Heat, and alſo keep it hot. In ten Minutes Ventilation it was perfectly cured of its ill Taſte; and after ſtanding twenty-four Hours in a broad Pan, there was a thick Scum which was half Cream and half Butter, free from any ill Taſte; the skimmed Milk was not ſheer or thin: So here is a Method to make good Butter from ill taſted Milk.

55. THE Froth of the Milk was ſo great, by reaſon of a too brisk Ventilation, as to make it froth over the Veſſel, which was thirty Inches deep; if it had not been kept down, by conſtantly lading and breaking the very large Bubbles of Froth. But when the Ventilation is more gentle, the Froth has riſen but three Inches from ſix Quarts of Milk, which was nine Inches deep. The Cabbage Milk was but ſix Inches deep. I repeated the like Operation the ſame Day, with the Evening Milk of the ſame Cow; but giving it only a Heat, that I could bear my Fingers in, for a little Time;

Time; with this Degree of Heat, after forty-five Minutes Ventilation, the Milk (tho' much better tasted) yet was not so compleatly cured, as the former Milk. Hence we see, how necessary Heat is, to volatilize the rancid Oyl (which gives the ill Taste) to such a Degree as to cause it to fly off by Ventilation

56. It was observed that what was milked from this Cow a Week after she had done eating the Cabbage, had an ill Taste.

57. I have not as yet had an Opportunity, to try to cure, in the same Manner, the ill Taste of Milk, which is occasioned by Cows feeding on autumnal Leaves, or Turnips, they having probably eaten this Autumn, the fewer Leaves, on account of the Plenty of Grass, occasioned by much Rain; which has also hitherto prevented Turnips from being rancid, which are observed to be most so, when they shoot out in the Spring. As Opportunities offer I purpose to make Trials, which I conclude others will also do, which will

probably

probably be attended with the same good Effects as that on the Cabbage Milk.

58. But tho' the ill Taste of Milk from feeding on Cabbage Leaves, was thus effectually cured by volatilizing with Heat, and dissipating by Ventilation the rancid Oil; yet the bitter Taste of a strong Infusion of Chamomel Flowers in six Quarts of Water, was not sensibly abated by an Hour's Ventilation of it, while scalding hot.

59. I am informed that, in *Devonshire*, they set the Pans of Milk on Trivets, making Fires under them, to give the Milk, gently and gradually a scalding, but not a boiling Heat, which would disturb the rising Cream; and then set it on the Floor in the Milk-house to cool, where in twelve Hours it has a thick Scum, partly Butter, and partly Cream: The skimmed Milk is very thin and sheer; and the Cream in great Plenty and delicious, except it gets a smoky Taste, which it is apt to do; and which might probably be prevented, by having a Range of as many Stoves, as

there are Pans of Milk to be used at one Time; all to be warmed by one Fire, either at one end, or the middle of the Flue or Funnel in the Brick-work, which conveys the Smoke and Heat under the Stoves, And as the Pans nearest to the Fire will soonest have their due Heat, on their Removal to bring the farthest and coolest Pans nearest the Fire; and instantly covering the uncovered Stoves with proper Covers to prevent the Heat and Smoke from coming out; by this Means the Milk would all be soon heated, with any kind of Fuel, and that with much less in Quantity than in the common Way.

60. AND the more effectually to prevent the Smoke from coming at the Milk, it may be well to have the broad outer Rim of the Pans turned perpendicularly downwards, three or four Inches, that it may enter deep into a circular Groove of Sand; and if it shall be needful the Sand may be wetted in order the more effectually to prevent the Passage of the Smoke: I thought of this Method about fifty Years since on tasting the smoky Butter in *Somersetshire*.

merfetfhire. By the fame Means the Poor might fave much Fuel in boiling the Pot, efpecially in Summer, when a Fire is wanted only for boiling the Pot.

61. WHEN any Pans are to be removed from the Stoves, the Afcent of the Smoke thro' the uncovered Stove, may be prevented by firft clofing the Flue near the Fire, by an Iron Sliding-fhutter or Regifter.

62. MILK might thus moft commodioufly be heated to a fcalding Heat with little Fuel, fit for Ventilation, in a Veffel of a proper Depth, fet in the fame Manner as the Pans in a Stove, to fecure it from Smoke, with Bellows fixed properly near it: (fee *Fig.* 3.) By this Means there would be little Trouble or Expence in curing ill tafted Milk by Ventilation.

63. *May* 14th, meerly to fee what the Event would be, a Gallon of new Milk, juft from the Cow was ventilated, for an Hour and half, which produced fix Ounces of Butter; and tho' it was ventilated half

an

an Hour longer, yet no more Butter was made; it was whitish, wanting both the Colour and Taste of good fresh Butter.

64. I am credibly informed, that in the Places famous for making the best fresh Winter Butter, they set the Pot of Cream in warm Water, so long as till it has acquired that small Degree of Sourness, which it very soon has in warm Summer Weather, which gives it its agreeable Flavour. And in order to give it Colour, they grate a well coloured Carrot into a little Milk, which as soon as stained, is strained from the Carrot thro' a Sive, and then mixed with the Cream.

65. It is found by Experience, that the Quantity of Cream is increased, by putting into the Milk a little warm Water in Winter, and cold in Summer; which being thereby, in some Degree thinned, the Cream is thereby more easily disintangled, so as more freely to ascend to the Surface of the Milk.

66. I ventilated three Gallons of ſtinking *Jeſſops-well* purging Water. On firſt blowing, the Smell of the aſcending Vapour was very offenſive, which Offenſiveneſs abated much in five Minutes: In eleven Minutes the Smell was much better: In twenty Minutes the Water ſeemed ſweet both in Smell and Taſte; and not ſweeter at the End of forty-five Minutes, fifteen or twenty Minutes will probably ſuffice.

67. *July* 20th three Gallons of ſtinking Sea-water were ventilated; in five Minutes it was much ſweetened, and no ill Smell in the aſcending Air, tho' at firſt it was very offenſive: At the End of ten Minutes it had a ſmall Degree of ill Taſte; after twenty Minutes no ill Taſte or Smell. It frothed near a Foot high during Part of the Ventilation; this from the Bitumen, *&c.*

68. Some Sea-water which was made to ſtink with Fleſh, and Iſinglaſs being put into it, was not made perfectly ſweet, not even

even by a ventilated Diſtillation, and an Hour's more Ventilation after it was diſtilled; ſo that Putrefaction with animal Subſtances, is not eaſily compleatly cured by Ventilation.

69. When the Water was 27 Inches deep in the leaden Veſſel, no Air could be blown up thro' it by the Force of the Bellows. But at 18 Inches Depth, the Air could freely be blown up in Showers thro' the Water; when therefore it is requiſite to blow up thro great Depths of Water, the Bellows may be worked with a Lever, as Smiths Bellows are worked.

70. As it is found by Experience, that the Milk and Butter of Cows, which drink ſtinking Water, has a very bad Taſte, this plainly ſhows that the Water retains its putrid Quality when mixed with the Blood; whence it is much to be ſuſpected, that the ſtinking Water which is drank in Ships, by retaining its putrid Quality, even when mixed with the Blood, may thereby promote that putrid

trid Distemper the Scurvy, as well as some other Distempers. And much more does the putrid close Air in Ships, which is mixed with the Blood from the Lungs, promote putrid and other Disorders: By the same Means also, pestilential Infections are taken in: For as the salutary Properties of good Air, are conveyed to the Blood by the Lungs, so are also the malignant Qualities of bad Air.

71. THUS also the putrid Water in marshy aguish Countries, may be a Cause of Agues, as well as the putrid Air which they breathe; which, as well as the putrid Water, may probably carry some of its putrid Quality into the Blood thro' the Lungs. This Method therefore of sweetening stinking Water, by blowing Showers of Air up thro' the stinking Water of some aguish Places, may be beneficial.

72. LIVE Fish may well be carried several Miles, by blowing now and then fresh Air up thro' the Water, without the Trouble of changing the Water; for this Ventilation will not only keep the Water
sweet,

sweet, but also enrich it with Air, which is necessary for the Life of Fishes; with which Air they supply their Blood, by breathing the Water, thin spread, between their Gills: But stinking Water will kill Fish.

73. I HAVE found that much of the heating Oil may be got out of Tar-water, by blowing Showers of Air up thro' it when scalding-hot, for 15 or 30 Minutes, the longer the better; the less volatile, and more salutary Acid remaining.

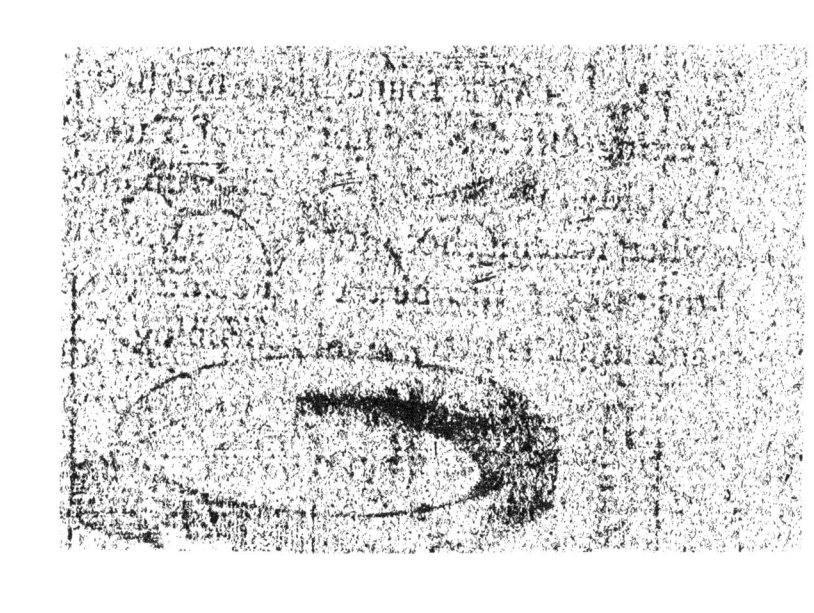

page 59

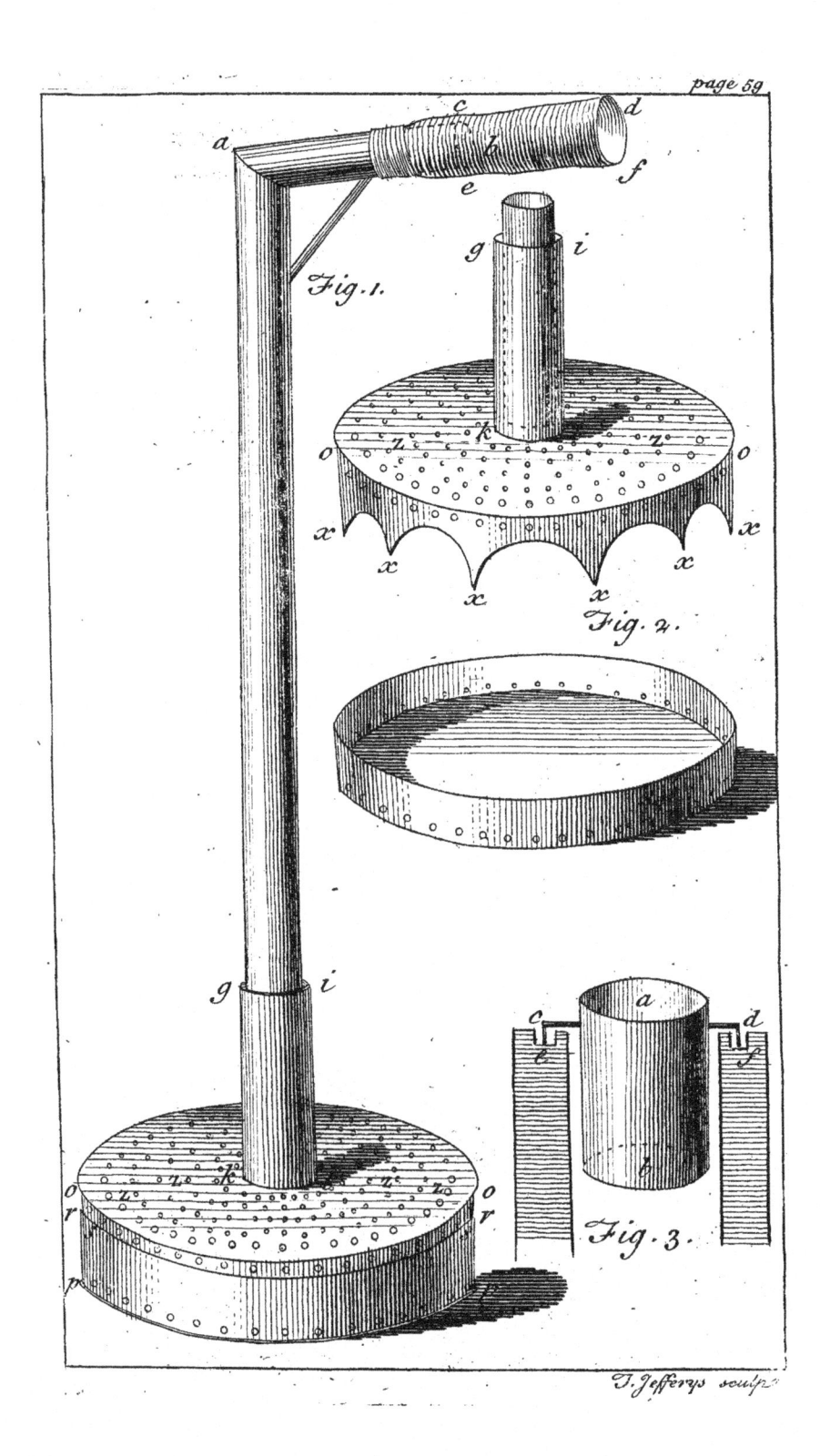

Fig. 1.

Fig. 2.

Fig. 3.

T. Jefferys sculp.

Explanation of the FIGURES.

Fig. 1. (o o p r) a Tin or Copper Air-box, six Inches Diameter, and an Inch and half deep from (o to p.)

The Lid of the Box full of Holes, one twentieth Inch Diameter, and about a quarter of an Inch distant from each other.

(g i k l) a Nozel soldered to the Lid of the Air-box, into which the Tin-pipe (a g i k l) is fixed so as to take in and out; this Pipe to be two Feet long, and six-tenths Inch Diameter.

(a b) a Bend in the Pipe five Inches long, to which is fastened the leathern Pipe (c c d f) six Inches long; to which the Nose of the Bellows is fixed at (d f.)

Fig. 2. (g i k l o o x x) the Lid of the Box, whose Rim (o x o x,) is a quarter of an Inch deeper than the Box (o p Fig. 1.) that the Air-holes (o) may be pierced in its Upper-part; and the Lower-part is scoloped with wide Scolops for the Air to pass through the Holes (p p Fig. 1.)

Fig. 3. (a b) the Milk-boiler, with the broad Rim (c d) and the perpendicular Rim (c e d f) soldered to the horizontal Rim; the perpendicular Rim to enter the circular Groove (e f) four Inches deep full of Sand, thereby to prevent the Ascent of the Smoak from the Fire Stove.

❀ ❀

BOOKS *written by the Rev.* STEPHEN HALES, *D.D. and printed for* R. Manby, *in the* Old-Bailey, *near* Ludgate-Hill.

I. Statical Essays in 2 vols, 8vo. The first containing an Account of some Statical Experiments on the Sap in Vegetables. The second, Hemestatics; or, an Account of some Hydraulic and Hydrostatical Experiments made on the Blood and Blood-Vessels of Animals.

II. Philosophical Experiments; containing useful and necessary Instructions for such as undertake long Voyages at Sea, 8vo.

III. A Description of Ventilators; whereby great Quantities of Fresh Air may with Ease be conveyed into Mines, Goals, Hospitals, Workhouses, and Ships, 8vo.

IV. An Account of some Experiments and Observations on Tar-Water; wherein is shewn the Quantity of Tar that is therein, and also a Method proposed to abate that Quantity considerably, and to ascertain the Strength of the Tar-Water, 8vo.

V. An Account of some Experiments and Observations on Mrs. *Stephens*'s Medicine for dissolving the Stone; wherein their dissolving Power is inquired into, and shewn, 8vo.

VI. Some Considerations on the Causes of Earthquakes; which were read before the Royal Society 1750, 8vo.

VII. *The Wisdom and Goodness of God in the Formation of Man:* Being a Sermon preached before the Royal College of Physicians, *London, Sept.* 21, 1751, 4to.